Your Sister Your Brother Your Neighbor Has AIDS

Your Sister Your Brother Your Neighbor Has AIDS

But wanting to justify himself, he asked Jesus,
"And who is my neighbor?"

Luke 10:29

Deborah Elandus Lake, M.Div.

Brush Arbor Press, Chicago

This book is not meant to be used to diagnose HIV, AIDS or any other disease or condition. The only way that you can know if you have HIV is through a medical test.

Published by Brush Arbor Press

Visit our website at *www.sankofaway.org* to learn more about our programs and services.

To purchase additional copies of this book:
email - sankofaway@sankofaway.org
voice - 773 624 5669 fax - 773 624 5689

Printed in the United States of America.

ISBN 13: 978-0-615-14269-2

Clinical consultant: Terri Pease, Ph.D.
Book design by Ellen Peace

All Bible verses are from the New Revised Standard Version (NRSV)

In memory of W. E.

Thank you for allowing me to be your companion

as you transitioned from this world.

Rest in peace.

PREFACE

The personal journey that led to me write this book started when I realized just how ignorant I was about the impact of HIV/AIDS in our communities. I was ignorant about AIDS as a disease. I was ignorant about how many of us are touched by HIV and AIDS. I was ignorant about how HIV/AIDS impacts people's emotional and spiritual wellbeing. Despite being a trained health care chaplain, I was totally uninformed about how to minister to people who were living with HIV/AIDS.

I thought HIV and AIDS were not part of my world. They were something people suffered with in the remote areas of Africa, or within the white gay male population. HIV/AIDS was something people got because they were careless, promiscuous, or uninformed. Since my daughters, my friends, my colleagues, and I were none of these things, I thought we were all immune to HIV infections. I believed that I only had to think about HIV/AIDS when and if I wanted.

As a seminary intern at Metropolitan Community Church in New York (MCC/NY), I occasionally encountered gay men and/or IV drug users who identified themselves as HIV positive. I also knew about the history of HIV/AIDS in America and the devastation the disease had caused in the lives of gay men. Despite these occasional pastoral encounters, and my historical knowledge, I did not understand the prevalence of HIV/AIDS in my world. I was a Black woman who had lived most of my adult life as a heterosexual. I had Black heterosexual daughters who were not abusing drugs and were not sexually promiscuous. In my mind, I was safe; my daughters were safe. Then, I went to The Ruth Rothstein CORE Center to work as an HIV/AIDS chaplain.

At the CORE Center, I encountered people infected with HIV who were from a variety of backgrounds, ethnicities, and sexual orientations. They had become infected with HIV in a variety of ways—some of whom believed they were in monogamous heterosexual relationships. Most of the people that I encountered at the center were Black. Many were heterosexual. Some even reminded me of people that I knew and loved.

PREFACE

Serving at the CORE Center as the chaplain brought HIV/AIDS into my world. I began to realize that no one was immune to HIV/AIDS. In response, I began to build an emotional wall between myself and my 'clients'. I concentrated on my clinical responsibilities—I made chart notes, completed intake forms, and documented my spiritual assessments. I was meticulous about charting my 'encounters' with my clients. I was diligent about completing my intake forms. I was almost obsessed with documenting my spiritual assessments. Before I began to provide pastoral care, I would complete my clinical responsibilities by asking a round of questions and checking the appropriate boxes. I had things under control. I kept a professional distance. I was headed down a path that many people take when facing difficult issues that remind them of their own human vulnerability until I met Trisha.

Trisha was a Black woman about 30 years old who had come to the CORE Center's women's clinic for years. The first time I met her I started my routine clinical responsibilities. In the middle of my usual round of assessment questions Trisha stopped me with a sharp question:

"Why do you need to know all this about me?"

Trisha wanted to know why I needed to know where she lived to take care of her spiritual needs. She wanted to know why I had to know how she became HIV positive to pray with her. She wanted to know what difference it made whether she was homeless or living with a family member in how I took care of her spiritual needs.

Trisha challenged me to justify why I put forms, assessments, and tracking questions ahead of her spiritual needs. She challenged me to see that I was treating her as though she were a statistic on the many reports my employer needed to complete to keep our funding. Her question prompted me to look her in her eyes and, for the first time, see her pain, anger, and confusion. For the first time, I did not push away my feelings by focusing on a form.

I was speechless and ashamed. I realized that I was becoming comfortable with hiding behind my clinical training to keep from facing the vulnerability of my clients and feeling the connection that we have as humans. Trisha made me stop and see her as a person. She made me stop putting reports between my clients and me. She made me begin to realize that she and I were not different.

That day, I stopped completing forms first. I stopped having "encounters with clients." I stopped tracking the demographics of clients first. That day, the day I was challenged, touched, and embarrassed by Trisha, I started the journey toward becoming an HIV/AIDS pastor. I was heading down the path of providing pastoral care without being emotionally available when God put Trisha in my way.

Because of Trisha, and her blunt questions that frightened, silenced, and shamed me into seeing her as a human being rather than a statistic, I started to minister from my own vulnerability and humanity.

Today I do not mentally separate people who are HIV negative from those who are positive. I do not trivialize the impact that having HIV/AIDS has on a person's life, but I understand that the disease touches everyone.

I hope that this book will help others avoid taking the same road that I first took. I hope that you can start out knowing that HIV/AIDS is a human condition that can only be addressed with human connection, empathy, and unity.

I learned years ago, early in my theological education, that I needed to be a global rather than a dogmatic pastor. People in need of spiritual care have concerns that fall outside what we normally consider Godly. Most of the times their concerns cannot be addressed through religious dogma. Simply telling someone to believe something is just not enough.

People are lonely, and sometimes believe that their loneliness is a punishment from God. People are abused by their loved ones, and often believe the abuse is God's Will. People struggle to keep their children out of trouble, and many times they believe that trouble comes from an angry God. Many are people who seldom attend church, and have very little patience with dogmatic sermons. Still, they need spiritual guidance. They want to feel as though they are connected to something greater than themselves.

To take this need seriously, I had to stretch beyond my Union Theological Seminary education. I had to see beyond my clinical training. I had to learn how to use what I knew as a theologian and a clinician to make bridges to address both the physical misery, the emotional discomfort and the spiritual distress people lived with daily. This meant that I had to learn about conditions that many pastors consider to be outside the church. I had to learn how to address matters like domestic violence, sexual assault, trauma, child abuse, and yes, HIV/AIDS.

In addition, when I began to focus on the concerns of people living with HIV/AIDS, I realized that I had to learn how to take care of physical misery, emotional discomfort, and spiritual distress in the context of living as a Black person. I had to learn how to care for and empower people who lived in a world that is at best indifferent and at worse, hostile. Because I found no 'experts' to show me how to care for the physical misery, emotional discomfort and spiritual distress of Black people living with HIV/AIDS, I became my own expert. I found ways to bring a spiritual connection to addressing the challenges people faced because of racism, misogyny, and homophobia.

This book is the result of a journey that began years ago with my learning, first from the people at the CORE Center, and later from many others, how to provide spiritual care that is authentic in Black communities while addressing HIV/AIDS. Most of what I learned came from listening to people who were living with HIV or AIDS. I learned from people who, despite the fact that their spiritual needs had consistently gone unmet, put their trust in me and shared their hopes and dreams. They taught me what they hoped for in a spiritual community and dreamed about a time when these hopes would be fulfilled.

The journey led me deep into my shortcomings. My journey put a spotlight on my bigotry. My journey took me to a place where I was able to cry along with my 'clients' and still be able to care for their needs first. I wrote this book to share what I have learned with caregivers, family members, and loved ones who support people living with HIV/AIDS. If I have been successful, this book will serve as a guide to ways to help stop the spread of HIV in our communities. It is not my intention to preach the 'right' way to be—God lets us all know what is right and wrong when we listen. It is not my intention to convert people to a particular way of maintaining a spiritual connection—only you can decide what personal spiritual path is best for you.

A special word to clergy: I have written this book for family members and other lay people who face the challenge of loving and caring for people affected by HIV/AIDS. But, it is my hope that pastors, chaplains and other professional religious helpers will find in these pages a guide to addressing HIV/AIDS in their daily work as well. This book is written in clear, every day language rather than professional jargon. And, because this is a book for the lay reader, you will not find a complex discussion of the theological underpinnings of this work. Instead, you will find information that can help you recognize the special spiritual concerns that arise in the context of HIV/AIDS care.

We do not need to talk about Thomas Aquinas and Christology, or grapple with Calvin's and Locke's understanding of soteriology[1] to recognize and meet the spiritual needs of people who are dealing with HIV/AIDS. To meet people where they are spiritually—to help them see their next step and take it—you need empathy, information about how HIV/AIDS affects people's spiritual and emotional lives, and guidance on how to recognize and address spiritual distress in an interfaith context. It is my hope that you will find what you need in this book.

---

[1] Christology and soteriology are terms theological scholars use to describe their studies of Christ, His life and salvation.

PREFACE

Whether you are a lay person, a pastor, a seminary student, a social worker, chaplain, or health care worker, *Your Sister Your Brother Your Neighbor Has AIDS* is your support as you learn how to care for the people in your life—your patient, your sister, your brother, your neighbor—with HIV/AIDS.

Reverend Deborah Elandus Lake, M.Div.

Acknowledgments

To those who read the many stages of this book:
    Thank you for your input and constructive criticism.

To my clients who made me the minister that I am today:
    Thank you for your trust.

To my daughters who never lost faith:
    Thank you for your encouragement and laughter.

To Terri for never giving up:
    Thank you for being my partner, no matter what.

To my ancestors for the sacrifices you made:
    Thank you for allowing me to be.

To God, all praise, honor, and glory.

Contents

INTRODUCTION

As spiritual people who overcome social, physical, legal, economical, and psychological challenges every day in our lives,
African Americans receive spiritual guidance and gain emotional
wisdom in many ways. We read the Bible or other sacred books,
attend religious services, meditate, pray, listen to or read the testimonies of others, and follow what we hear in our hearts.

We receive guidance from listening to or reading about people
who have overcome the same challenges that we are facing, and
our spirits are fortified because we no longer feel abandoned. We
gain wisdom from listening to or reading about people who
shared their feelings, thoughts, and reactions as they overcame

the same challenges that we are facing, and our emotions are soothed because we no longer feel helpless.

Spiritual guidance and emotional wisdom are part of every day life for us. They come with our connection to one another. They come when we are in relationship with one another. When spiritual guidance and emotional wisdom are left out of our lives, we feel cut off from a major source of strength and comfort. Cut off in this way, we are not unlike the man near death who was lying in the road after being robbed and beaten. We need a neighbor to care.

As African Americans who are living with HIV/AIDS, our sisters, brothers, and neighbors[2] not only face the same challenges that we all have in day-to-day life, they also face the social, physical, legal, economical, and psychological challenges that come in a life with HIV/AIDS. Our sisters, brothers, and neighbors make decisions that reflect their spiritual distress—their feeling of being isolated, insignificant and separated from God. They express feelings that reveal their emotional discomfort. While there is a great deal of information available on how to understand and help address the social, physical, legal, economical, and psychological challenges that come with

---

[2] Our sisters, brothers, and neighbors with HIV/AIDS are of different and even changing genders. However, our language makes it difficult to reflect that fact in writing. In this book I will use the pronouns he/him and she/her interchangeably—any *her* could also mean *him*—any *he* could also mean *she*.

HIV/AIDS, there is very little *non-denominational* guidance on how to understand and help address spiritual distress and emotional discomfort.

HIV/AIDS present particular spiritual and emotional challenges. Often these challenges are illustrated through the questions people express and the feelings they experience. For instance, questions arise that reflect the stigma some denominations place on our God-given sexuality. Feelings of extreme guilt are commonly linked with these questions. People ask "why did God let this happen to me?" while feeling that they deserve to be punished. In other words, they blame God for *letting* them get HIV and at the same time, they believe that they deserve what they have gotten.

In many people's minds, HIV transmission is closely connected to sexual activity. Religious teachings may criticize any sex outside heterosexual marriage, and most condemn homosexuality outright. Because of this, we often believe that those living with HIV/AIDS are somehow spiritually flawed or that they are being punished for past behavior. People who are living with HIV/AIDS often believe the same thing about themselves. This is why many of us are in disbelief when we learn that someone who lives inside our theological backyard has been infected with HIV. This is also why part of our own process of accepting that someone we know and care about is HIV positive includes questioning how such a terrible thing could have happened.

In *Your Sister Your Brother Your Neighbor Has AIDS,* I have created a guide to help you learn to care for the person you know who is facing challenges to their spiritual and emotional well being because of HIV/AIDS. It does not matter whether a person is your partner, your spouse, your child, or your friend—like the Good Samaritan, you know that person is your neighbor.

I have included verses from the Bible to help you understand six stages of experience that people often go through as they respond to learning that they have HIV or AIDS. As you read, remember:

- *Your Sister Your Brother Your Neighbor Has AIDS* is your chance to 'walk in the shoes' of someone else.
- The feelings, thoughts, and reactions that are described in the six stages give you an overall view of what it is like when a person learns that he or she has HIV or AIDS.
- *Your Sister Your Brother Your Neighbor Has AIDS* also gives you guidance on how to take the next step—helping your neighbor incorporate having HIV or AIDS into a healthy lifestyle.

I have also included several sections that will be a resource to you while you help your neighbor:

INTRODUCTION

- At the beginning of each chapter you will find a prayer. I wrote these prayers to help you focus on a particular challenge and to ask God for help.

- At the end of each chapter you will find a testimony. The testimonies are from people who are either living with or who know people living with HIV or AIDS. Their stories are real. Details have been changed to protect their privacy.

- Every chapter has a *Make It Real* section. I included this space for you to keep track of your feelings, thoughts, and emotions. Remember that you may write about feelings that are private, so treat the *Make It Real* sections as though they are part of your journal.

In addition to information to help you help your neighbor, *Your Sister Your Brother Your Neighbor Has AIDS* also has information to help you. I have included basic information on how you can center yourself and stay centered.

While HIV and AIDS are life-threatening and cannot be cured, people go on to live healthy and productive lives for ten, fifteen, twenty years or more after testing positive for HIV. The main thoughts to hold dear as you learn to be a support to your neighbor are:

- While having HIV or AIDS changes a person's life, the change does not need to mean that all life is over.

- Many people overcome the emotional impact of a diagnosis of HIV or AIDS and find new ways to be productive in their communities and inspirational to the people that they meet. While details have been changed to protect the privacy of individuals, you will learn about some of these people when you read the *Your Neighbor Speaks* sections.

Whether you are HIV positive yourself, or not, thinking about HIV and AIDS will set you on an emotional and powerful journey:

- When you read and track your thoughts and feelings you will be changed.
- The fact that you are reading this book means that you already have concern for people living with HIV or AIDS. Once you have finished, your concern will be reinforced with knowledge.
- After you have read *Your Sister Your Brother Your Neighbor Has AIDS*, you will be able to support your neighbor with HIV or AIDS and you will be able to encourage your neighbor to seek more help.
- The fact that you are starting this journey means that you already see a need for change in yourself and in your neighbor. Once you have finished, the need for change that you now see will be replaced with practical actions.

INTRODUCTION

A word of caution: as you learn how to relax and become centered, you may discover feelings, thoughts, and memories you did not know you had. Some of these feelings, thoughts, and memories can be the result of old hurts and painful events in the past. These feelings, thoughts, and memories may interfere at times when you need to focus on important matters in your daily routine. If this is the case over a period of time, do not hesitate to seek professional help. In the resource section of this book you will find a list to help you get started.

So, let's begin. Find a safe space for yourself. This is the place, in your home or somewhere else, where you feel safe and will not be easily interrupted by others. Your safe space should be comfortable, accessible, and familiar. Once there, stay in the moment and pay attention to your feelings.

You may be afraid of what you will learn. Maybe you feel you are going against God's Will by learning about HIV/AIDS. Perhaps you are angry. Or, you may simply be curious. Whatever your feelings are, try to pay attention to them while you are in your safe space. You will find spaces to write some of your feelings down in this book. If you have a favorite Bible scripture or quote, keep it near. Read it often. Then, when you are ready, begin your journey. And always remember,
God is with us.

Your neighbor
  a man in his early 20's
speaks:

I was infected in jail, I think. I have been gay for as long as I can remember, but I never told anyone because I knew they wouldn't understand.

All through school, I had girlfriends because I didn't want anyone to know that I liked guys. I got one girl pregnant. We thought about getting married, but that never worked out. I was going to church back then because she wanted us to. I didn't like it because I knew the preacher there liked guys. He had approached me, but I don't do preachers.

The first time I had sex with a guy I was 15. He was 20. Before that I'd just messed around a little, but mostly just thought about being with guys. He took me to his house, and I spent the night with him. The next day I went home and we never saw each other again. After that I would go to gay bars to let men pick me up and take me home. A lot of times I'd have sex in the bathroom with several guys during the night.

I was also on the party circuit where old men would have weekend parties in their houses for other old men who wanted to have sex with young guys like me. They had a lot of money and sometimes one of them would buy me clothes, or drugs, or give me some money. It was fun when one of them would let me drive their car. I did a lot of drugs then—mostly Meth.

I was still trying to have a relationship with my baby's mother. We would have sex off and on, but that wasn't going too good. She was getting tired of me disappearing for days at a time, and was asking too many questions.

I was 19 when I got arrested for selling drugs. Since it was my second time being in trouble, the judge gave me time. While I was there I was raped by several guys. I came out with HIV. I don't know if I had HIV when I went in, or if I got it while I was there.

I worry about my baby's mother, and I am still trying to figure out how to tell her that I have HIV. She would kill me if she found out that I have been with men. She hates fags, and she would think I was one if she knew. I know that I have to tell her, but I can't. I am trying to get her to get tested, though. My counselor told me that I can encourage her to get tested without telling her that I have been with men.

1

Getting Ready

Y ou are about to start a life-changing journey that will give you:

- Basic information about HIV.
- The ability to identify some of your neighbor's needs.
- Guidance on how access HIV/AIDS resources.
- Information to help you stay centered.

Chapter One, *Getting Ready*, gives you basic facts about HIV/AIDS, and important information about acute and chronic illnesses. Use this information as you learn to become a helper to someone with HIV or AIDS. In this chapter your main goals are:

- Keep yourself open to new, even frightening, information.
- Remember that God is your source of strength and courage.
- Stay with the spiritual routines that you already have.

Let's start with a prayer:

A prayer for readiness

Prayer is talking to God. Prayer is praising the Almighty, asking our Higher Power for something. Prayer is a way of acknowledging that we are connected to the Divine.

Prepare My Heart

God, You are all-powerful. You are all-knowing. You are greater than any one person, institution, organization, or group. Your Will is beyond all understanding.

Prepare my heart as I prepare to learn.

God, You have no need, yet You are the source! All that I am, all that I will be, all that I cherish, comes from You. You have no deficit, yet through You all change occurs! My transformation, my knowledge, my wisdom, are engendered by You.
I thank You!

Thank You for the past and present blessings. Thank You for the blessings You will give in the future.

Prepare my heart as I prepare to learn.

Today God, I will begin to learn about something that is frightening. I am going to read about a disease that has no cure. This disease has taken many lives. In my human condition, I have feelings.

I am afraid.

> *I have fear, but I know that Your Strength is with me.*

I am uncertain.

> *I have doubt, but I know that Your Wisdom will guide me.*

I am sad.

> *I have sorrow, but I know that Your Presence will comfort me.*

I am bewildered.

> *I have confusion, but I know that Your Word will free me. You will fortify my soul, my mind, and my body so that I will be able to do what needs to be done. I know all these things through faith. I ask all these things in the name of Jesus Christ. Prepare my heart as I prepare to learn,*

Amen.

HIV is a virus - AIDS is a disease

We often talk about HIV and AIDS together, as though they are the same thing. HIV and AIDS are connected, but they are not the same. A person can have HIV but not have AIDS. Here are some things that we know:

- We know that HIV is passed from person to person through intimate interactions that involve body fluid-to-body fluid contact.

- We know that there is no vaccine to protect us from getting HIV and no cure for AIDS.

- We know that everyone who develops AIDS is also infected with HIV.

HIV is the nickname of a virus. The full name is *Human Immunodeficiency Virus*. Not everyone with HIV is sick with AIDS. HIV can live in a person's body for a long time—maybe even years—before they get sick with AIDS. Anyone with HIV—sick or well—can pass the virus on to others. The only way to know if you or someone else has HIV is through a medical test.

Outside of the body, HIV cannot live. HIV is not passed from person to person through ordinary touching, hand shaking, sharing towels, forks or spoons, or from a kiss on the cheek. Friends pass on HIV by sharing needles used for drugs, tattoos or piercing. Lovers pass on HIV by having unprotected sex. Mothers

4

pass on HIV during childbirth or while breast-feeding. AIDS is not passed on from person to person. AIDS develops after a person has been infected with HIV.

There is no vaccine to protect us from with HIV.

AIDS is the nickname of a serious disease. The full name is *Acquired Immune Deficiency Syndrome*. This name says that the body is not able to protect itself from other dangerous germs. Most people's bodies fight off germs easily. People with AIDS cannot fight off germs. They get sick.

There is no cure for AIDS.

About Acute and Chronic Illnesses

Some illnesses only last a short time. We call them *acute* illnesses. We can get a cold, an infection or even something dangerous like appendicitis, get medical care and become completely well. Other illnesses cannot be cured or they last a long time. We call them *chronic* illnesses.

Diabetes and sickle cell are examples of chronic illnesses. Medicine, proper care, and diet can help people feel better and lead healthier lives. But there is no cure.

AIDS is a chronic illness. It will not go away, it cannot be cured.

New medicines are making a difference. Some medicines help people with HIV to stay healthy. They can avoid developing AIDS for years. After a person develops AIDS, medicines help them fight off germs. This helps them stay well. But even with the best medicines, a person can still pass on HIV.

When helping your neighbor, remember that living with a chronic illness is difficult:

- People want to believe that they are not really sick.
- They may feel angry, sad, and hopeless.
- They may avoid seeing a doctor or taking medicines that have powerful side effects.
- If their medicine helps them feel better, they sometimes think they are cured.

As you help a person with HIV or AIDS, keep in mind that these are normal reactions that come with having any chronic illness.

About Helping

If you are planning to take care of a loved one who has HIV or AIDS it is important to take care of yourself too. Helping people is difficult work. Helping people we love and care about is even more difficult.

GETTING READY

Our emotions are strong when we know someone personally. We have a history with the person. If you are helping a family member, spouse, or partner, you may not be able to imagine life without your loved one.

Such strong feelings can cloud our judgment and cause us to make decisions that are harmful. We may become overwhelmed with our own emotions. There are precautions you can take to avoid this, and there are steps you can take to find your way out of feeling overwhelmed. The rest of this book will give you information to help your loved one with HIV or AIDS and information for taking care of yourself as well. Remember that you have chosen to do something that is extremely difficult.

First, know that deciding to help someone living with HIV or AIDS is a commitment to a rocky road of ups and downs, of trips to the hospital, of pain, loss, and grief. Your decision to help means that you will be changed for life, and with change always comes discomfort.

You will also experience joy and freedom. You will have the joy that comes with helping someone survive and overcome troubled times. You will experience the freedom and power that come when we work to develop an open and grateful spirit.

Second, remember that you cannot do or be everything for your neighbor or loved one. There are resources that you can use, and people who are available to help you help your neighbor. Do not wait to ask for help for yourself. You may even want to schedule regular time with a professional when you can focus on your feelings, thoughts, and needs.

Third, remember that it is okay to say, "I can't do that." Just as there are resources for you, there are even more resources for your neighbor. While resources differ from state to state, overall we are fortunate in the United States because people with HIV or AIDS have access to medical care, social services, psychiatric care, and medication. When your neighbor's needs are beyond your ability to help, the best action you can take is to make sure that she gets the help that is there.

Fourth, remember to take care of your needs. We can spell the word *new* with the letters N U and E to remember how to keep well. Remember to *Nourish yourself*. Remember to *Unwind* with friends or a hobby. Remember to *Exercise*. Keeping N-U-E in mind will help you keep new/nue and refreshed.

Nourishment is key to having and maintaining a strong body and mind. The old saying, "you are what you eat" is true. If you skip meals, load up on caffeine, and eat more meat than fruit and vegetables, you will eventually suffer physically and mentally.

GETTING READY

Having and maintaining healthy eating habits is not only important for you, this is important for your neighbor as well. By
eating well, you will be a valuable example.

Unwind with friends, family, and loved ones regularly. If you do
not have a hobby, this may be the time to start one. The time that
you set aside to play, reconnect with friends, and feel joy in your
life will keep your spirits uplifted and your expectations optimis-
tic. This is especially important because HIV/AIDS takes over a
person's life. Often, the illness is all a person living with HIV or
AIDS can see or think about. You will need to be able to bring
freshness into your neighbor's life, and the best way to do this is
to consistently renew/nue yourself.

Exercise is important to having and maintaining a healthy and
flexible body. You will find that as you become more involved
with helping your neighbor, regular exercise can be one way to
keep your focus and your perspective. In addition, exercise will
help you sleep. There will be many nights when you will be unable to sleep because of events you experienced with your
neighbor. A good workout, jog, walk, or weightlifting routine
will help you get relaxed enough to fall asleep easily.

Remember that the *Make It Real* pages in this book are an important part of your self-care plan. Take the time to keep aware
of your own feelings. Write down ideas and plans that will help

you care for yourself and your loved one. Also remember that you may want to keep this section private.

Make It Real

Who are the resource people in my life who can help me as I help a person with HIV or AIDS?

Is there a group I'd like to join, an activity I'd like to try?

How do I comfort myself now?

What time will I save just for myself today?

2

Steps to Understanding

This chapter will make it easier to understand how to help someone who is living with HIV or AIDS. Think of these six steps as stepping-stones. Each one leads you down a path that many people with HIV or AIDS have followed on their way to a new sense of dignity, love, and self-respect.

This chapter describes thoughts, feelings, and reactions that people commonly experience when they are going through the process of incorporating HIV or AIDS into their lives. Read this chapter so that you, the helper, will be able to 'walk in these shoes' in a small way.

In Chapter Two, *Steps to Understanding* your main goals are to:

- Learn about the fear people have when they find out they have HIV or AIDS.

- Learn about how that fear may paralyze them or cause them to 'act out' in particular ways.
- Learn about feelings of loss, regret, and blame.

This chapter may be especially difficult for you to read. You may even find that some of your own feelings come forward. If this is the case, there is information about self-care in this book that will be very helpful for you.

Remember to use the *Make It Real* section as a way to help yourself process what you have learned and to get in touch with your feelings. Let's continue with another prayer:

STEPS TO UNDERSTANDING

A prayer for humility and wisdom

Prayer is talking to God. Prayer is praising the Almighty, asking our Higher Power for something. Prayer is a way of acknowledging that we are connected to the Divine. Prayer and contemplation help us open ourselves to change when we know that there is nothing we can do to change things. Prayer and contemplation are power. With prayerful contemplation, comes wisdom and humility.

Lead Me to Understanding

Almighty, all knowing, and loving God, all praise belongs to You. All thanks belong to You. You are all powerful and the source of all the knowledge and wisdom that I have.

It is through You, that I have dignity, humanity, compassion, and love.

I thank You for being my Creator, and for guiding me in life. Give me the wisdom that I need to be able to make the necessary changes in my life.

Give me the humility to know that I am a work in progress, and will continue to learn and grow for as long as I live.

God, You care for my needs even before I know how to call them out. I have needs today. I have feelings today.

I am in agony.

> *I anguish over what could have been. I anguish over mistakes I think I have made. I anguish over what might come to be.*

I am in fear.

> *I am afraid of the future. I am afraid of pain. I am afraid of rejection. I am afraid of isolation. I am afraid that I am condemned.*

But even as I cry out, I know that, with You I will prevail. I know that, with You, I have strength. I know that with You, I have peace.

Guide me as I begin to learn about what it means to live with HIV and AIDS. Give me your wisdom as I help my neighbor make crucial decisions. Give me the courage to ask for help and the ability to accept help when it comes. Bring only people who are Your instruments into my life.

Keep destructive feelings like anger, hatred, and helplessness out of my heart.

Keep destructive states like drunkenness, promiscuity, and deception out of my mind.

STEPS TO UNDERSTANDING

Keep destructive people like homophobes, racists, and pessimists out of my life.

For even though HIV and AIDS are life threatening, the spirit never dies. We all live on with You, through You, and in You. Continue to give me what we need to do what I have to do. Continue to show me how to do the work You would have me do.

It is in the name of Jesus, the healer, the teacher, the forgiver that I pray,
Amen.

STEP One—The News

Terrors are turned upon me; my honor is pursued as by the wind,
and my prosperity has passed away like a cloud. And now my
soul is poured out within me; the days of affliction have
taken hold of me.

Job 30:15-16

News about HIV/AIDS blows into your life like a winter wind:

- You visited your son in the hospital and learned that he had been HIV positive for a year.
- Your daughter found out she had AIDS as she delivered her first child.
- You accidentally saw HIV medicine in a friend's home.
- A family member just 'wanted to talk.'

No matter how the news came to you, it was unexpected. Now, you may have very strong feelings, many questions, and no idea about what the future holds.

Maybe you have noticed that your son's health has not been what it was. You remember the vibrant, strong infant that you brought into this world. You see glimpses of the inquisitive young child that you helped grow into manhood. You have watched your strong young man begin to waste and become weak. You are shocked when you see that his strength and vigor are gone.

Or, you are beginning to think about the fact that at the time your daughter is facing the responsibilities of motherhood she is also facing a life with AIDS. Your new grandson is facing the possibility of losing his mother. Your daughter is not going to be the mother that she could have been because of AIDS. As you process this, maybe your mind wanders back to when she first told you she was pregnant. You remember a happy young woman telling you her joyous news. You want that young woman back as you watch her asleep in her bed.

As you think about HIV and AIDS and start to help your neighbor, strong and surprising emotions may come up. It seems that at the very time when you need to save your energy for helping your loved one, you recall your own life story.

This can bring many strong and distracting feelings. It is very important to recognize your feelings, whatever they are. As you think about the changes you are facing, you may be flooded with memories. You may start to remember things that happened to you years ago. You may feel as though endless days of affliction are upon you. You may even feel that God has abandoned you and your loved one.

Sometimes these thoughts and feelings come all at once and without notice. You may find that you are crying 'for no reason' or have little interest in everyday activities. Such feelings may come when you are alone, on a crowded bus, at work, or on a busy street. Whenever your feelings come, it is important to remember these things:

- Your feelings might come at a time when it is not safe for you to let them show. It is okay to put off recognizing them until you are in a safe place with safe people.

- Your feelings can help you begin to heal from old hurts. The healing process may be very difficult, but it is worth the trouble.

- Your feelings may lead to more old memories and more old feelings. You may need to talk to a psychologist or counselor who is trained to help people work through traumatic experiences from the past.

You may think that it is better to ignore your own worries and pay attention to the person who is sick with HIV or AIDS. But it turns out that keeping a balance is better. Paying attention to your own feelings will actually give you more energy and greater compassion for others.

In addition, knowing how you feel about something means that you will be less likely to confuse your responses with your neighbor's. This will free you so that you can be less judgmental when your neighbor has a response with which you disagree.

Your neighbor
    a 36-year-old father and husband
speaks:

I couldn't believe that I had AIDS. I thought it must be a mistake. I wasn't supposed to get this. AIDS was for people who did wrong things. I was straight. I was a father. I had a job and had gone to college. I helped people who had these kinds of things.

At first, I went into denial. I didn't think. Didn't want to talk to anyone. I yelled at my kids so much that they avoided me. Now they are afraid of me. I started to hit my wife. She was tested and came back negative. I hated her for that.

I started to drink too much, and to hang out with the wrong people. I lost my job, most of my friends, and my family. It wasn't until I was home-less and looking to get a bed in a shelter that I cried for the first time.

I cried all that night in the shelter, and most of the next day. I had a mental collapse and had to be admitted into the psych ward on suicide watch. I had to learn that I was no different than anyone else, and that this disease does not just attack people who have no worth or who do things they shouldn't.

If there is one thing that I want people to learn from my life experience it is not to judge. I realized that I judged people a lot before, and I was wrong.

Most people want to do what is right, and they want to help others. I thought that only bad people got this disease and I lost everything I had because of how I thought. I had to start from scratch and start to build a life with AIDS.

Make It Real

Right now, I am feeling

I am afraid that later I might feel

The one thing that 'blows me away' is

I am sad because I have lost

STEP Two—Devastation and Loss

My eye has grown dim from grief, and all my members are like a
shadow.

Job 17:7

When first diagnosed with HIV or AIDS, your neighbor or loved one will begin a challenging and frightening journey. People with HIV or AIDS need your help and support. They need you to accompany them on their journey. Your neighbor or loved one may feel as though the world has been destroyed. HIV/AIDS are all she will think about. A person with HIV or AIDS may wonder if family and friends will reject them. Everything looks and feels different. It seems that life is over. A diagnosis of HIV/AIDS scatters any sense of what is familiar and comfortable. Eyes become dim from grief, and all one can see is sadness.

For instance, your son may have been preparing to go back to college when he learned he was HIV positive. His life, as you both knew it, has stopped. Now, the future you both looked forward to has been changed. Now, you both wonder about how he will get the medical care that he needs. Instead of thinking about college, he may only be able to think about what he fears may never be.

Or, your daughter was thinking about buying her first home before she learned she had AIDS. The future you and your daughter thought she might have is no longer in immediate reach. Now, you are concerned about how she will care for a new baby and get the medical help that she needs. Her life, as you both knew it, has stopped. Instead of enjoying her accomplishment of bringing new life into the world, she may only be able to worry that she will not watch her son grow into adulthood. You have a place in this process.

Your job is to both validate fear *and* hold on to hope. Your job is to have the wisdom to look through eyes that are dim from grief, *and* hold on to visions that are beyond the immediate sadness. You can do this by listening first. Listen to what your neighbor believes will happen. Encourage her to be in touch with her feelings, and not try to push them away. At the same time, encourage her to be in the moment. This will help her not become overwhelmed with thoughts of what might happen months or years in the future.

As you learn how to be in your moment and how to validate your own feelings, you will be better able to help your neighbor do the same. Encourage them to think about times when they overcame obstacles that they thought were insurmountable. Help them remember that they have your support, and help them recognize the support they have in their friends, loved ones, and

26

professional caregivers. Do not be afraid of your neighbor's sadness. Do not be afraid to let your sadness show.

While you are supporting your neighbor at the beginning of the journey you will take together, it is important to remember these things:

- It is okay to be sad and to mourn the loss of a life free of a chronic illness.
- If sadness stops you from doing what needs to be done, it is okay to seek the help of a mental health professional.
- Develop and maintain your personal relationship with God.

Your neighbor
   the pastor of a Pentecostal church
speaks:

I can no longer be silent. As a pastor of a church, I have seen several of my members die from AIDS. They were gay and they never talked about who they were. I lost too many people to this disease, and I can't be quiet any longer.

My tradition teaches that homosexuality is a sin, but the people that I know who died of AIDS were good people. They were people who tried to do what was right. After we lost them, I made a commitment to learn what I needed to know to take care of them and to help stop this disease from spreading.

It really doesn't matter what two adults do in their bedrooms.

It does matter that we are dying of AIDS, and it doesn't seem to be letting up.

It matters that children are losing their mothers and fathers and parents are losing their sons and daughters.

It matters that wives are getting AIDS from their husbands.

It matters that we are not doing everything we possibly can to stop the spread of AIDS.

Make It Real

The loss that is most on my mind today is

The fear that is most in my heart right now is

I feel that I have lost touch with

I can overcome being "dim from grief" by

STEP Three—Regret and Blame Take Over

My heart is in anguish within me, the terrors of death have fallen

upon me. Fear and trembling come upon me, and horror

overwhelms me and I say, oh that I had wings like a dove! I

would fly away and be at rest .

Psalm 55:4-7a

People living with HIV or AIDS often look for ways to make sense of what has happened to them. They may blame themselves. They may blame someone else. They may even believe that God is punishing them for past behavior. You can help during this time by reminding them that anyone can be infected with HIV. The virus does not seek out people who are evil and skip those who are good. Having HIV or AIDS is not a reflection of a person's spiritual or personal worthiness. To help your neighbor hold on to this fact, you have to believe it yourself. Ask God for the wisdom you need to evaluate what you truly believe about HIV/AIDS and God.

The sense of devastation leaves people feeling numb, isolated, and broken. It seems as though nothing will improve. They feel that they will always be outside and alone. They may start to relive every terrible thing that has happened to them. During this time they will search for reassurance and stability.

A great deal of regret, and a search for answers, may be a reaction that your neighbor or loved one has in response to HIV/AIDS. *How did this happen? My life has been stolen! I want to escape this nightmare!* They ask *why?* You may ask *why?* Your neighbor or loved one may lash out in anger against family, friends, even you.

If they are in recovery, there is a strong chance that they may use again as a way to fly away from this life-changing illness. Under strong pressure we all tend to rely on old behavior from the past. Using illegal drugs or misusing alcohol again at this time could be your neighbor's effort to regain some sense of control by returning to what is familiar.

For instance, your son may become withdrawn and not want to see you or any of his friends. He may refuse to talk about his feelings, and attack anyone who tries to help. Your son's doctors are concerned because he will not co-operate or even talk with them. They are worried that his ten-month recovery from illegal use of methamphetamine is in jeopardy.

You may be angry and afraid. You may be angry with him for taking chances with his future. You may be angry because the fight to keep him off drugs may be starting all over again. You may be afraid of your anger.

You may be afraid that you will say something or do something that will hurt him because you are so angry. If you find that you are feeling afraid and angry, it is important that you recognize this. Know that your response and your son's response are normal.

Or, your daughter does not want to hold her new baby. When you visit her, she is always in bed with her back to the door. When she does look at you, you can see that her eyes are swollen from crying. She looks as though she hasn't slept in weeks. She has lost more weight than she should over the last few months, and her sister is concerned that she is not eating. You notice empty beer bottles in her room and around her apartment.

Your daughter does not seem angry, but she refuses to talk about how she feels. She will not read any of the literature on AIDS that came home with her from the hospital. She will not discuss making plans for her first visit to her AIDS doctor. It is as though she is just waiting for death to fall upon her.

You find that you are focusing more on her baby and less on her. You may look forward to seeing your new grandson more than your daughter. Perhaps you find that you are feeling resigned and overwhelmed. You are resigned to the possibility that you will lose your child to AIDS and you are overwhelmed with your feelings of loss and sadness. For you and your daughter, it is important to recognize your feelings and know that your response and your daughter's response are normal.

You have a place in this process. Your job is to:

- Remain steady. Try to develop a routine. You can visit at the same time every day or week. If you cannot visit, you can call at the same time. This will give your daughter something to look forward to all while she believes that she has nothing.

- Talk with professionals. There is a great deal of help for family members of people who are living with HIV or AIDS. Use the resources in your area. Contact some of the national resources listed in the back of this book.

- Do not be afraid to talk with a person with HIV/AIDS even when he does not respond. He will hear you; he will take in what you say. You can give him hope and help him begin to see beyond the anguish in his heart.

While you are supporting your neighbor or loved one at this point it is important to remember these things:

- Stay in touch with your own feelings. You will get more information on how to do this as you read about prayer and meditation.

- Stay in touch with your HIV/AIDS resources. Read the literature that is available and use the help that you have.

STEPS TO UNDERSTANDING

- Stay in touch with your neighbor. Keep consistent contact
  with him neighbor and be the stability that he needs right
  now.

Your neighbor

A 25-year-old male-to-female trans person

speaks:

People need to know that God is for everybody. God doesn't just love you if you belong to the right church, or live a certain way. God is for everybody, and I want people to know that all they have to do is reach out and God will take their hand and lead them to people who are able to support them.

I remember when I first found out that I had HIV. I didn't care about myself. I used drugs, and did all kinds of things because I believed that God didn't care. Now, I know that 's not true.

I got sick and had to go to the hospital. They thought I was going to die. I had to slow down and start to accept the help that was there for me. I had to think about my life and how I got where I was.

There were people who talked with me and listened to me, and I found God again. I saw God in the people who helped me accept that I am HIV positive, and learn that I can build a life that is worth living.

Make It Real

Today, I want to "fly away" because

Safe ways to "fly away" for short times are

Unsafe ways to "fly away" might include

I most feel at rest when

STEP Four—First Things First

So do not worry about tomorrow, for tomorrow will bring wor-
ries of its own. Today's trouble is enough for today.

Matthew 6:34

Although HIV/AIDS does change things forever, there is still time to make decisions and learn about this new way of living. It is important to focus on what can be done in the moment, the hour, the day, rather than think about problems that may come in the future. Living with HIV/AIDS brings many problems, and the potential for more in the future. You can help by focusing on what can be done today and reminding your neighbor to trust that God will provide for tomorrow.

Once the reality of HIV or AIDS sinks in, it is hard to know where to start. Remember that there are three major things you can help with right away:

- Get accurate, unbiased information.
- Find the right doctor.
- Connect with the right support people.

With the diagnosis of HIV or AIDS, life changes. There is a great deal of work to do. Needs and problems may seem to be overwhelming. You can help by reminding your neighbor to focus on one task at a time.

For instance, your friend who has AIDS medication in his cabinet may be jumping from one topic to another while you talk. He may be overly concerned about the troubles that he reads about or sees on the television. You may notice that he has started to hoard things like canned goods, or toilet paper. This may confuse and irritate you.

You are confused about what to do after seeing the medication. Did he send you to get something from the cabinet so that you would see the medication? Is this his way of letting you know that he has AIDS? Should you tell your friend what you think?

You may also be irritated with your friend's behavior—he has not been straightforward with you. You are irritated because he did not trust you enough to tell you. You are irritated because you do not like not knowing what to do or say. That's okay. Remember that your friend's response is normal and so is yours.

Maybe your family member who just wanted to talk has now told you that she has HIV. It has been a few weeks, and you have not talked about it since then. You have noticed, though, that she stays away from bad news and says she can't watch the news or read the paper because it is too depressing and scary. Her house, always neat and clean in the past, is becoming more and more disorderly. She does not appear to be as concerned about her personal appearance as she was before. Her nails are chipped and broken. It looks as though she has missed several of her weekly trips to the hairdresser. She still goes to work, and takes care of her family, but there are small differences that let you know she is not feeling like herself. You may be surprised and disappointed.

You are surprised because you have never seen your family member lose control. She has always been the orderly person in the family. She was the person everyone could count on to have the right answer, or know the right number to call when things need to be done.

You are disappointed because you are confronted with your family member's humanity. Perhaps she is your older sister, and she has been the one person you always admired and wanted to imitate. It is a big disappointment to see her seem to slowly lose control of her life.

Or, maybe she is your mother and the person you have always believed would be there for you in times of trouble. Her diagnosis reminds you that she will not always be there for you. Understand that these reactions are normal so that you can do your job in this process:

- Identify your own feelings and reactions. As long as you do not identify your reactions, there is a strong chance that your feelings will get in the way of your being able to help.

- Remember that your loved one's behavior is probably temporary and is the best way they have in the moment to handle what they are feeling, thinking, and fearing. Do not judge with your words or actions.

- Let them know that you have noticed the difference and ask how you can help. Then, listen to what they say. Often people can identify the help that they need if someone encourages them to stop and think. If you ask the specific question—*how can I help?*—that may be the one thing that will allow a person to stop and think.

- If things continue to get worse, do not be afraid to suggest to your neighbor or loved one that they see a psychologist or counselor. Do not overreact, but be aware that things could get worse, and that a person may think about hurting herself or someone else. This is not something you can handle, so get professional help.

Your neighbor

a husband, father, and minister

speaks:

I was infected when I had unprotected sex with a prostitute while I was away at a convention. It was just one time. I came to be tested when I started feeling sick.

I felt so guilty after I had been with the prostitute. I had a feeling that I was going to get AIDS. So, I wasn't surprised when the test came back positive.

I had to figure out how to protect my wife, tell my children, and get my wife tested. It was very difficult because I was also the pastor of a church. I told my wife and she got tested.

I lost my wife and my church. Some of my children won't speak to me. For so long, I tried to be the perfect person. Everyone saw me as some-one who never did wrong.

My congregation didn't want to know that I struggled with problems or had doubts. My wife didn't want to know that I was struggling with my own mortality, and that every time I looked at her I was reminded of the fact that I am getting old. I tried to be perfect, and in the process did a very stupid thing.

For a long time, I hated myself. I even thought about killing myself. I didn't believe that I deserved to live. I believed that God had turned His back on me. Now I know that during this time, I still believed that I was supposed to be perfect. I couldn't forgive myself because I still believed that I should have been better, and not had the same problems and fears that ordinary people have.

Now, I realize that I am just like everyone else. Even when I was the pastor of a church, I was no different than anyone else. I had, and have, fears. I had, and have, problems. I had, and have, weaknesses. The difference now is I know this. I pray to God not to feel better about myself, but to gain wisdom and strength so that I can be the best person that I can.

I try to live my life in a way that makes it meaningful for others. That's why I thought it was important to give this testimony. I hope that when people read it, they will realize that they are not perfect and they never will be perfect. The best they can hope for is if they become the person that God meant for them to be.

Make It Real

New worries that we didn't have before are

The worries we need to take care of today are

Worries that may be imaginary are

Worries that I need help with are

STEP Five—Building a Support Network

Call to me and I will answer you, and I will tell you great and
hidden things that you have not known.

Jeremiah 33:3

God's work can be seen in the dedicated scientists, doctors, nurses, and counselors who have devoted their time and talents to the field of HIV/AIDS prevention and care. Before you began to read this book you may not have known that there are many advances in treatment, and that there are services and programs available for people living with HIV/AIDS. There is new research and ongoing development of protocols, programs, and medicines all the time.

You can help your neighbor or loved one remember that there is help available, and you can encourage him to utilize all of their resources. HIV/AIDS patients need to learn about what medications work for them. They need to take their medication as directed by their doctor.

The newer HIV/AIDS medications often involve complicated directions and schedules to work properly. The person who takes these medicines must have regular checkups and blood work. It usually takes several tries to find the right combination of medications.

The side effects of HIV/AIDS medications can be uncomfortable and frightening. They can change the way a person looks, feels and behaves. It takes a lot of trust between the person, their loved ones and the medical professionals who help them to get through this period. Still with the right combination of medicines many people with HIV/AIDS begin to live comfortable and satisfying lives.

It takes strength and courage to put up with making so many trips to the doctor and dealing with unpredictable side effects. Emotions can even get in the way of doing what has to be done. If this happens a person will need to find the right therapist, spiritual leader, psychologist, or psychiatrist. If they are addicted, they will need to work closely with their sponsor or find the right program to get help.

For instance, your son is getting better now, and he is beginning to address his anger. He thinks HIV was passed to him from his girlfriend, and most of his anger is directed toward her. He finally agreed to see a psychologist, and you can see a difference in him.

At the same time, you have been exploring your anger and may have discovered pain from your own childhood hurts. With both of you working through your anger, you have been able to have important conversations about your feelings.

Or, after your daughter was diagnosed as being clinically depressed, she got the psychiatric help that she needed. She is now on medication and sees a psychiatrist twice a week. She never really connected with her son the way you would have liked, but she now takes care of herself, and is taking her AIDS medication.

She was admitted into the hospital twice, but for the last six months she has been healthy. She is talking about looking for a job. You are encouraged, especially because you know she has stopped drinking. You feel more connected to your daughter now, and are enjoying your grandson who is almost two years old.

Your neighbor

a 53 year old wife and mother

speaks:

I was infected by my husband. Many people don't know who infected them, but I do.

I learned that I might have HIV when I found out that my husband had a girlfriend. The girlfriend had died of AIDS. I got tested and I had AIDS. I was devastated and could not believe what had happened.

It was a very hard time in my life and I was glad that I had my church. They didn't know, and they still don't know that I have AIDS, but being able to go there and pray helps a lot. I was able to forgive my husband, which is very important. I couldn't carry around a lot of anger and still do what I needed to do to stay healthy.

My husband is dead now. I was with him when he died. I took care of him for as long as I could. Now I have dedicated my life to teaching women that they are at risk for getting HIV or AIDS even if they have been married for 50 years. I teach women to take care of themselves, especially Black women, because we tend to take care of everyone else before we think about ourselves. I want my life to be an example of how to care about yourself and others.

Make It Real

Changes that I see in myself are

Changes I notice in my neighbor or loved one are

God has sent us help and information through

I see God's loving hand at work in

STEP Six—Deciding to Live With HIV/AIDS

We do not live to ourselves, and we do not die to ourselves. If we live, we live to the Lord, and if we die, we die to the Lord: so then, whether we live or whether we die, we are the Lord's.

Romans 14:7-8

The person with HIV/AIDS faces the challenge of making a decision to live. Living on means more than taking medication, eating and sleeping well, and staying sober. It also means:

- Being responsible and loving.
- Deciding to live a healthy life.
- Determining who should know and when they should be told.
- Discovering how HIV/AIDS fits in an ongoing life story.

Once people know that they can live on, they will want to have friends and relationships again. With this they will need to be responsible and loving friends, partners, spouses, parents and family members. This is the time to make the conscious choice to live a healthy life. A healthy life includes making good decisions about when and how to be sexually active with another person, and when to talk about one's HIV status. With help, your neighbor will learn how to incorporate their HIV status into an ongoing life. They will find communities that build self-respect and treat them as human beings.

Deciding to live on with HIV/AIDS does not mean becoming resigned to illness, familiar with isolation, and overshadowed by death. Living on means living a better, healthier life. Living on means continuing to be active members of society. Living on means accepting life's joys and blessings with gratitude and humility. Living on means knowing that sometimes God sends help through unknown people at least expected times.

Your neighbor

a father in his forties

speaks:

I made mistakes in the past, and that's part of why I'm here today with this disease. But, I also have knowledge that I can teach, and that's what I want my life to be about. I want to teach people what I have learned so that they won't have to live through the same mistakes that I have.

I want my life to be worth something. If I have this disease, it will be worth living if I can just stop one person from making a mistake that will change the rest of his life.

Make It Real

Something that I know now that I did not know before

is

Next steps that I will need to take myself are

Other places my neighbor can find help include

To feel valuable to my neighbor I need

3

Keeping Strong

When Jesus went into the desert before He began His ministry, He went into the desert to fast and pray in solitude (Matthew 4:1-2). Before His betrayal, arrest, and crucifixion, He went alone into the garden to pray (Luke 22:39-44). He prayed for strength to do what God wanted Him to do. He also accepted the things He could not change in His life, and asked God to guide Him through the troubled times He was facing.

You too can follow the example left by Jesus in your every day life. You can identify what you already do to keep yourself relaxed and centered. You can also explore new ways to become relaxed and centered. If you feel that you do not know how, this book can help you build a daily, weekly, or monthly routine to relax and find your personal center. Let's continue with another prayer:

A prayer of freedom and gratitude

Prayer is talking to God. Prayer is praising the Almighty, asking our Higher Power for something. Prayer is a way of acknowledging that we are connected to the Divine. Prayer and meditation are ways that we open ourselves to the universe. Prayer and meditation are ways that we accept the power that is ours for the asking. Prayer and meditation are ways we can comfort ourselves. With prayerful meditation comes a free and grateful spirit.

Give Me the Strength to Know My Weakness

God, I thank You for the journey I have taken. Thank You for Your guidance and thank You for the helpful people You have put into my life.

While You are the source of everything, there are some parts of my life that are under my control.

It is up to me to free my heart from envy, anger, and dishonesty. It is up to me to redirect my mind so that I am grateful for everything that I have been given in the past and all that I have right now.

I will be looking into myself even more as I learn how to include meditation with prayers to you. Just as Your Son went into the desert to pray, fast, and meditate, so will I learn to be still and know.

Help me see where I have been blinded by my pride.
Help me recognize where I fall short of who and what You want me to be. Help me know if my feelings and emotions are becoming too much for me to bear alone,
Amen.

Keeping Your Center

We all have times in our lives when we feel off balance. These are the times when we feel as though everything we do only makes things worse. Or, we may feel as though there is nothing that we can do and that we are powerless to make things better. During times like this, people say they feel abandoned by God. Others describe having a wall between themselves and the rest of the world. Some say they cannot pray. Feelings of having lost all ability to help, or having lost the support of people who care are very common.

Chances are you have overcome serious stress in the past. Take a moment to remember your personal successes in times of stress. Let this memory give you the confidence to face the present challenge.

Besides knowing your own strength, and your past successes, you can remember to stay centered and take time to relax. During times of stress and confusion taking a moment lets you see beyond your immediate problems and feelings of isolation. Self-reflection is crucial to understanding your personal reactions to events. Self-reflection is also an important aspect of being able to recognize when you are biased or favor a particular perception over another. Recognizing your bias will be important when you talk with someone who is living with HIV or AIDS and has a lifestyle or belief that is different or in contradiction to yours. There are some specific things you can do, to "take a moment" in the face of the stresses and worries you experience in being a neighbor to a person with HIV or AIDS. Be sure to pay attention to your own comfort, get centered and breathe. Take time to notice your own reactions, and even to write down your thoughts and feelings.

Write: Writing can be a very helpful tool as you begin the relaxation and centering part of this process. By writing down your feelings, thoughts, and impressions, you will be able to track how you feel in connection to particular people, memories, and events. This will be important information as you engage in self-reflection and examination while fulfilling your role as helper.

Comfort: It is important to have a consistent way of calming yourself. You can use any hobby, chore, or activity that comforts you. If you find yourself getting comfort from activities that make you feel embarrassed, guilty, or that cause you emotional or physical pain afterward, you will not achieve your goal of becoming relaxed and centered. In fact, you may have the opposite result and find that you are more tense than before.

Center: Being centered means that you are able to be still. When you are centered this means that you have a sense of yourself and the rest of the world. You are connected to the rest of the world, but you are also aware that you are separate.

Relax: Relaxing is a physical and mental process. You will need to be in touch with your body and feel when your muscles are tense and when they are becoming less tense. Many of us carry tension in our backs and necks. The expression of the tension is pain and stiffness in our necks and backs. Be aware of this and ask someone you know to massage your neck and back, or even consider getting a professional massage. This will give you a chance to learn where you carry your tension if you do not already know.

Breathe: Breathing is important in the process of becoming relaxed and centered. Your breathing should be deep, slow, and regular. Over the period of a week try to pay attention to your breathing as you go about your regular day. Try to write down when you notice changes in your breathing. Also write down what you were doing when the change happened and who was with you.

Wait, Watch, Listen: If you can, try to take time to be alone in a quiet place. Turn off the radio, television, and any other distraction and take a few minutes to sit quietly and wait. Write down any thoughts, memories, feelings, or impressions that you have during this time. From time to time, go back and read what you have written and look for patterns and themes that may be present.

Make It Real

I have learned to center myself by

When I take time to breathe, I notice

I have found strength in

Today I know this about my neighbor and my-

self

Afterword

Next Steps

Now you are ready to help. You can be a companion to your
neighbor because you have taken the time and effort to become
acquainted with some of the feelings, thoughts, and reactions
that come with a diagnosis of HIV or AIDS.

Like the Good Samaritan, you care. Now, you have the basic information that you will need to act:

- You know the difference between acute and chronic ill-
  nesses.
- You know some general reactions to expect from a person
  who is living with a chronic illness.
- You know about the basic difference between HIV and
  AIDS.

- You have basic information about how HIV is passed from one person to another.
- You know about the importance of self-care.

Reading this book has allowed you to walk in your neighbor's shoes:

- You have more insight to behavior you may encounter as you help your neighbor adjust and live on.
- You have more understanding about why your neighbor may seem unable to get help on her own.
- You are more able to recognize the difference between your reactions and the reactions of your neighbor.

The sections called *Your Neighbor Speaks* have broadened your view of who is affected by HIV or AIDS. You now know that HIV/AIDS touches everyone regardless of income, profession, age, orientation, or gender. You also know that people can live on after learning that they have HIV or AIDS.

Now that you have a basic understanding of what it means to live with HIV or AIDS, there is a great deal of help you can offer your neighbor:

- You can help your neighbor identify medical, social, and legal resources.

- You can help your neighbor think through legal decisions including who will have medical power of attorney and who will have guardianship of minors.
- There will be a great deal of information, new people, and appointments that your neighbor will need to remember. You can help with this by encouraging your neighbor to start a daily log and contact book.

This is the time for you to put what you know into action. At the end of this book there is a resource section. If you have not already done so, make sure to look through this resource list. In addition to these national resources, look for ones that are in your area and write them down in this book. Looking for local resources and beginning to develop your own circle of support is the next step after following the instructions in this book. The SWSSinc website, *www.sankofaway.org*, may have links to resources in your area.

Reading this book was your first step. You needed to walk in your neighbor's shoes. You needed understanding. Your next steps should lead to empowerment:

- Empower your neighbor by encouraging him to develop a list of local resources and important people.
- Empower your neighbor by encouraging her to keep track of appointments.

- Empower your neighbor by encouraging him to think about and take care of legal concerns before there is an emergency.

Remember that you have been a powerful influence in your neighbor's life. Also remember, not everyone will be able to return and thank you for being there for them (Luke 17:11-19). Take comfort in knowing that you followed the teaching of Jesus when he shared the story of the Good Samaritan who took up the burden of his neighbor until his neighbor was able to care for himself.

RESOURCES

The information in this section is not meant to represent all of the resources that are available for people with HIV or AIDS and their friends, families and loved ones. Your city, state, county or tribal department of health may also be a resource for services in your community.

The Centers For Disease Control and Prevention (CDC)
> A source for general health information and specific information about HIV/AIDS transmission, prevention and HIV/AIDS funding.

website **www.cdc.gov/hiv**
telephone number **(800) 458-5231**

Sankofa Way Spiritual Services, Inc. (SWSSinc)
> A non-profit organization that offers information about supporting people with HIV/AIDS, training for professionals on HIV/AIDS and spiritual care and leadership in community education within Black communities.

website **www.sankofaway.org**
telephone number **(773) 793-5211**

US DHHS Substance Abuse and Mental Health Services Administration (SAMHSA)
> An agency of the U.S. Federal government that provides information about mental health and substance abuse.

website **www.samhsa.gov**

RESOURCES

The Body
>A comprehensive website with extensive information about HIV/AIDS care, medication medical care and prevention.

website **www.thebody.com**

Gay Men's Health Crisis AIDS Hotline
>A hotline operated by a community-based organization committed to national leadership in the fight against AIDS. Provides crisis HIV/AIDS support for all people impacted by HIV/AIDS. Callers do not have to give their names.

telephone number **(800) 243-7692**
TTY for deaf callers **(212) 645-7470**

National Domestic Violence Hotline
>A toll-free number to call from anywhere in the country to access safety from abusive relationships.

website **www.ndvh.org**
telephone number **(800) 799-7233**

OTHER RESOURCES

_____

_____

_____

_____

_____

_____

_____

_____

_____

_____

_____

OTHER RESOURCES

_____

_____

_____

_____

_____

_____

_____

_____

_____

_____

_____

About the Author

Reverend Deborah Elandus Lake is the founder and Executive Director of *Sankofa Way Spiritual Services, Inc.*, (SWSSinc) a non-profit, faith-based organization that searches the past for lessons and wisdom to make a better future.

Before 2004, when she made a full-time commitment to developing SWSSinc, Lake was a chaplain at the Ruth Rothstein CORE Center in Illinois where she provided spiritual care to people living with HIV and AIDS and their families. She was also a chaplain at RUSH University Medical Center in Illinois and Bay State Hospital in Massachusetts where she cared for the spiritual needs of people living with mental illness and trauma.

Reverend Lake is a graduate of Union Theological Seminary in New York, has two years of Clinical Pastoral Education (CPE) training, is a trained National Organization for Victims Assistance (NOVA) counselor, a Red Cross HIV/AIDS instructor, and has addressed the spiritual, emotional, and social needs of people living with trauma, illness and exclusion for over ten years.

To contact Rev. Lake or for more information about SWSSinc programs and publications visit our website: www.sankofaway.org or email: sankofaway@sankofaway.org.

www.ingramcontent.com/pod-product-compliance
Lightning Source LLC
Chambersburg PA
CBHW022029090426
42739CB00006BA/345